How I Lost Over 30 Pounds

And Counting...

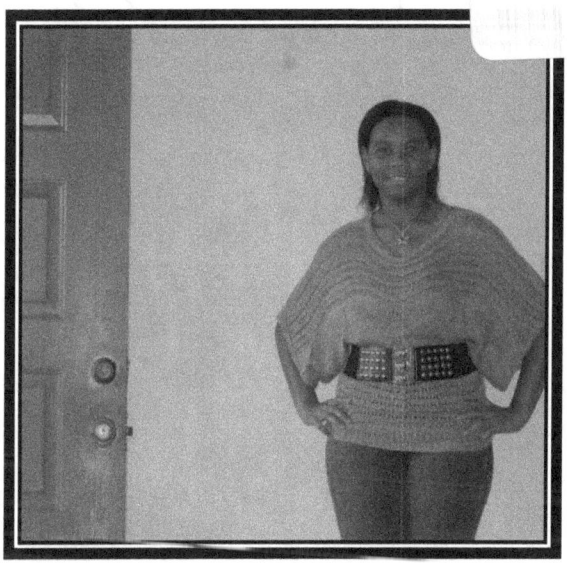

By Alicia Jasmine Faulk

Table of Contents

Introduction

I have struggled with my weight ever since I could remember. When I was little, I always had a bigger stomach, thighs, arms, etc. than the other girls my age. Even though I was made fun of in grade school, I was fortunate enough for it to stop before middle school.

In middle school I was treated better, but the damage was already done. Then and now, I remember the taunts. I became increasingly unhappy with my appearance. In eighth grade, I was at my heaviest: 198 pounds. I was 14 and 5ft 1in. That meant that I was obese, and headed down a dangerous path. In the future, I could have diabetes, heart disease, and/or other issues possibly leading to an early death. But, to me, the worst part was that I didn't want to look in the mirror or go out in public. And even worse than that, was that I didn't want family to see my ballooning weight.

I was in third grade when my mom first put me on a diet. I lost at least 20 pounds, but I didn't want to be forced to do it; so I quit and gained more weight.

My mom wants me to be a capable adult, and as I got older, she let me do more and more, eventually letting me choose what I eat. This was the single most helpful thing to my weight-loss. I felt like I was in control! I would just write what I wanted on the shopping list and she would buy it.

When it comes to losing weight, you have to have determination, motivation, and a want to better your life. Your reasons have to be good enough to make you commit to it, not do it now and quit later. Sure, an upcoming reunion or vacation might get you motivated to lose a few pounds, but losing weight and keeping it off is a lifestyle change.

Trial and Error

Some people will lose weight just by reducing portions. Some people will just by exercising. Others, it will take both. But there are some, like me, will need trial and error to find out what works for them. To lose weight, I needed a high protein diet that had more protein than carbohydrates. Losing weight takes patience and an understanding of your body enough to find what works.

Step 1: Stop Making Excuses

The title is pretty explanatory. The number one reason why people don't choose to lose weight, or even try to, is because of excuses. Excuses like: *I can't find a gym, Eating right is expensive, A gym membership is expensive, I have kids, I have a busy schedule, I'm a student, etc.* are holding you back from achieving your goals. There are simple solutions to these excuses:

I can't find a gym- You don't need one

A gym membership is expensive- Again, you don't need one

I have kids- Get them involved or exercise when they sleep

I have a busy schedule- turn errands into your exercise

Once you stop making excuses and make a plan, you can finally begin this process. I made many too, but the excuse making has to stop.

Step 2: Realization

Weight loss is a **lifestyle change** that only **you** can chose to follow. No one else can make that decision for you, and you can't make that decision for anyone else. The first step is to realization is to know what you're eating and how much. The best thing to do is to go in the kitchen and look through the fridge, freezer, and pantry for unhealthy food. Get rid of it and keep the healthy food. You need to look at your food's nutrition facts; I cannot stress this enough. Just because something says that it's healthy doesn't mean that it is. You need to look at a few things when deciding if something is healthy enough to eat: *Is it baked/ boiled/ or fried? How many calories are in it? How many carbs are in it? How much fat is in it? What kind of fat? How much sugar is in it? How much sodium is in it? What are the ingredients?* These questions need to be seriously considered before buying something.

Next, realize that eating right will cost more money than eating wrong.

Then, you have to realize that there is no secret or mystery to losing weight. There is no miracle pill to help you lose weight. Eating right and exercise is the only way to not only lose weight, but to keep it off too. Weight loss isn't easy.

Step 3: Get Motivated

Getting motivated will help you stick with your plan. This isn't about other people, it's about **you**. A good start would be to write down on a piece of paper what you want out of this. For example, your realistic goal weight, all that you want to do, no matter how far out there it is, and your reasons. I'll start: 135-140 lbs, wear a bikini, tank top, shorts above the knee, live a long life, and like the image the mirror shows me.

Step 4: Start Out Small

Losing weight and keeping it off is a lifelong commitment. You can't just quit once you get to your goal weight, you have to stick with it. Starting out small is the best way to ease the transition to a healthier life.

- Find out what you're eating, and how much
- Keep a food journal before and after you start
- Portion control
  - Buy smaller plates so you put less food on it; you can get seconds if you're still hungry
- Don't drink soda, sweet tea, etc.
  - Water is the best choice because your body needs it and it isn't filled with empty calories (calories that don't fill you up)
- Try to incorporate more exercise into your life
  - Walk or bike to work (if it's safe and/or not a very long distance)
  - Take the stairs (or take some of them if you work on like the 7th floor and up)
  - Exercise in front of the TV or computer
  - When you go to the store, park further from the store to walk more

Step 5: Eat Right

This is the most important step of weight loss. You need portion control. You need to eat slower to feel for when you're full and stop eating. **The food serving sizes on this plan and the number of snacks can be modified to fit your individual hunger.**

You can look at the nutrition facts of fruits and vegetables by looking on www.caloriecount.com, www.calorieking.com, or www.produceoasis.com for foods you either eat or want to try. You can modify the serving sizes, brands, or whatever to suit your individual needs.

Breakfast

Option 1: 2 ½ slices of turkey bacon, 1/2 banana with 1/8 cup of berries (I eat blueberries)

About 150.4 calories, 14.2 fat, 16.1g carbs and 6.2 grams of protein

Option 2: Special K Protein Plus cereal (With optional fruit) with Hood milk

About 170 calories, 7.5g fat, 17g carbs, and 15g protein

Option 3: Quaker Old Fashioned Oats Oatmeal (With optional nuts)

About 220 calories, 7.5g fat, 30g carbs, 10g protein

Snack

Model 1: Jolly Time popcorn without butter

About 20 calories, 0g fat, 5g carbs, <1g protein

Model 2: Pure Protein Bar (Chocolate Chip, Chocolate Deluxe, and Peanut Butter)

About 200 calories, 5g fat, 18g carbs, 20g protein

Model 3: 100 Calorie Pack

About 100 calories, 3g fat, 17 carbs, 2g protein

Model 4: 1 piece of Whole wheat bread with fat free cream cheese

About

Model 5: Apple slices with fat free cream cheese

Lunch

Model 1: 4 slices of turkey bacon and 1 clementine

About 175 calories, 12.1g fat, 8.9g carbs, 8.6g protein

Model 2: Progresso Light Soup

About 60 calories, 1g fat, 12g carbs, 3g protein

Model 3: Spinach, crushed almonds (1 ½ Tbsp.), and light dressing (I eat fat free Italian)

About 101 calories, 7g fat, 7g carbs, 4g protein

Dinner

Model 1: Tuna (Recipe in back) with a small salad

Model 2: 1 Chicken breast, vegetables, and a vegetable or zucchini pancake or a shrimp eggroll

Model 3: 1 chicken breast and steamed (or boiled) vegetables

This is what my school-time day looks like

Breakfast

Egg/ egg white mix

2 slices of turkey bacon

Fruit

Snack

½ a serving of vanilla Chobani yogurt

Diced peaches packed in water fruit cup

1(or less) serving of veggie straws

Lunch

Rotisserie chicken sandwich meat

Reduced fat Sargento pepper jack cheese

1 sandwich round

Fruit (or vegetables)

Step 6: Exercise

Exercise is essential to not only lose weight, but also to help keep it off.

Legs

1. Standing side leg raises

2. Laying side leg raises

3. Donkey leg raises

4. Knee raises

5. Laying down knee raises

6. Cycling

Stomach

1. Crunches
2. Weighted sit ups with dumbbells
3. Side crunches
4. The plank

Arms

If you have very little time for exercise I recommend Shawn T's T25 program

Step 7: Keep it off

This new lifestyle is forever. You can't just lose the weight and go back to old ways.

Staying Motivated

Staying motivated and away from stress is the hardest part. When I began writing this book, I had lost 55 pounds. But now, near the end of writing, I gained 30 pounds and lost 10. I gained the weight because I had a very stressful junior year and lost some of my motivation. I'm going to lose this last 20 and then some, and keep it off.

Keeping your motivation

Tips

Recipes

Mango Smoothie

½ a mango

½ a lime

Crushed ice

A little water

1 packet of Truvia

Directions: Mix together the mango, lime, water, and Truvia in a blender. Then blend in the ice.

About 53.5 calories, 0.2 g fat, 14 g carbs, and 1.4 g protein

Grapefruit Smoothie

½ grapefruit

½ lime

Crushed ice

Little water

1 packet of Truvia

Directions: Mix the grapefruit, lime, water, and Truvia with a blender. Then mix in the ice.

About 41 calories, 0.1 g fat, 13.3g carbs, and 1.8 g protein

Shirataki Seafood Delight

1 bag Shirataki noodles

Shrimp and scallops

Whatever vegetables you like

Teriyaki or soy sauce

Directions: Wash and boil the noodles. While the noodles are boiling, cook the shrimp and scallops in a pan and cut the vegetables if they need cutting. Add the teriyaki or soy sauce to the seafood. When the seafood is cooked, add the vegetables to it and teriyaki or soy sauce if you'd like. You could add optional egg whites for an extra protein boost. Drain the noodles when they're ready and mix them with the seafood and vegetables.

About 200 calories, 2.5 g fat, 3g carbs, and 38 g protein (without vegetables)

Add 75 calories, .75g fat, 17g carbs, and 1.5g protein for ¼ cup brown rice

Shirataki With Chicken

1 bag shirataki noodles

2 medium or 3 small Chicken breasts

Whatever vegetables you like

Liquid egg whites (optional)

Teriyaki or soy sauce

Directions: Wash and boil the noodles in a pot. While the noodles are boiling, cut the chicken, and the vegetables if they need cutting. Cook the chicken first with whatever seasonings you want and add some teriyaki or soy sauce. When the chicken is almost done cooking but not raw, add the vegetables in. After the vegetables are done, you can add the optional liquid egg whites for an extra protein boost. Drain the noodles and mix in the chicken and vegetables.

About 235 calories, 5g fat, 2g carbs, 47g protein

Add 75 calories, .75g fat, 17g carbs, and 1.5g protein for ¼ cup brown rice

Tuna

This recipe serves about 1-2 people and is high in fat; eat this only twice a month.

1 can of canned tuna

Light mayonnaise

Relish (optional)

2 whole eggs

Directions: Boil the eggs in a pot. While the eggs are boiling, mix the tuna, relish, and light mayonnaise in a bowl. After the eggs are done, peel them and chop 1 egg into the tuna mix. You can eat the egg white of the last one and chop the yolk into the tuna, or eat the yolk. You can eat crackers with it.

About 365 calories, 22.5g fat, 10g carbs, 32g protein

Green Bean Casserol

Feeds a lot of people and is good for parties. Divide it as small as you want because it is very filling. **(Not my own recipe)**

1 can cream of mushroom soup

2 cans green beans (drained)

¾ cup milk

Dash of black pepper

3tbsp. French fried onions

Directions: Mix the soup, milk and pepper into a bowl. When mixed, add the drained green beans. Put the contents of the bowl into a pan, add the onions on top, and put it into the oven however long it needs to cook.

The whole thing is about 415 calories, 18.5g fat, 46.5g carbs, 13.5g protein

Freezer Pops

Crystal light or another flavored water mix you like (has to be zero or close to zero calories, sugars, carbs, etc.)

A packet of Truvia (optional)

Freezer pop molds (I see them in Walmart)

Directions: It's best to make a full pitcher of the drink and poor it into the molds. Put the molds in the freezer for a few hours. Since it is zero everything, or at least very low, you can have as much as you want. Having the full pitcher is great because you can refill the molds as you eat them.

Baked BBQ Chicken

This recipe serves 1 person, and can be grilled instead of baked.

1 chicken breast or serving size of wings

Whatever seasonings you like

BBQ sauce

Directions: Season the chicken and put it in the oven. I like to put a little teriyaki sauce on it with the seasonings. When the chicken is almost fully cooked, add the BBQ sauce and let it finish cooking.

About 110 calories, 2.5g fat, 0g carbs, and 23g protein

List of Foods

Some of these measurements may differ by the kind or brand you buy.

- *Progresso* light soups (Zesty! South Western-Style Vegetable Soup)
  - Serving size: ½ can; 60 calories, 1g fat, 12g carbs, 3g protein
- Turkey Bacon
  - Serving size: 1 slice; 35 calories, 3g fat, 0g carbs, 2g protein
- Light Mayo
  - Serving size: 1 Tbs.; 35 calories, 3.5g fat, 1g carbs, 0g protein
- Sweet Relish
  - Serving size: 1 Tbsp.; 20 calories, 0g fat, 5g carbs, 0g protein
- *I Can't Believe It's Not Butter!* Original
  - Serving size: 1Tbsp.; 70 calories, 8g fat, 0g carbs, 0g protein
- *Hood* Calorie Countdown Milk
  - Serving size: 1 cup; 70 calories, 4.5g fat, 3g carbs, 5g protein
- Chicken Breast
  - Serving size: 4oz or 1 breast; 110 calories, 2.5g fat, 0g carbs, 23g protein
- Shrimp
  - Serving size: 3oz; 100 calories, 1.5g fat, 0g carbs, 21g protein
- Scallops
  - Serving size:1/2 cup; 100 calories, 1g fat, 3g carbs, 17g protein
- Broccoli
  - Serving size: 1 1/4 cup frozen; 20 calories, 0g fat, 4g carbs, 2g protein
- Wild Salmon Fillets
  - Serving size: 4oz or 1 fillet; 100 calories, 2.5g fat, 0g carbs, 19g protein

- *Jolly Time* White High in Fiber Popcorn Kernels (Air popped)(Can have more)
    - Serving size: 2 Tbsp. unpopped; 20 calories, 0g fat, 5g carbs, <1g protein
- Canned Tuna (I get Starkist Chunk Light)
    - Serving size: 1 can; 100 calories, 2g fat, <2g carbs, 20g protein

- Brown Rice
    - Serving size: ¼ cup; 75 calories, 0.75g fat, 17g carbs, 1.5g protein
- *Pure Protein* Bars (Chocolate chip)
    - Serving size: 1 bar; 200 calories, 5g fat, 18g carbs, 20g protein
- *Special K* Protein Plus Cereal
    - Serving size: ¾ cup; 120 calories, 1g fat, 19g carbs, 10g protein
- *Quaker* Old Fashioned Oats
    - Serving size: ½ cup; 150 calories, 3g fat, 27g carbs, 5g protein
- Cream of Mushroom soup
    - Serving size: ½ can; 70 calories, 2.5g fat, 10g carbs, 1g protein
- Canned Green Beans (Fresh and Frozen also options)
    - Serving size: ½ can; 20 calories, 0g fat, 4g carbs, 1g protein
- Canned Peas (Fresh and Frozen also options)
    - Serving size: ½ can; 60 calories,0.5 fat, 10g carbs, 4g protein
- Canned Collard Greens(Fresh and Frozen)
    - Serving size: about ½ cup; 60 calories, 2g fat, 6g carbs, 3g protein
- Teriyaki or Soy Sauce
    - Serving size: 1 Tbsp., can use a little more; 15 calories, 0g fat, 2g carbs, 1g protein
- *Kellog's* Original Rice Krispies Treats

- o Serving size: 1 bar; 90 calories, 2g fat, 17g carbs, >1g protein

- Liquid Egg Whites

  - o Serving size: 3 Tbsp.; 25 calories, 0g fat, 1g carbs, 5g protein

- French Fried Onions

  - o Serving size: 2 Tbsp.; 45 calories, 3.5g fat, 3g carbs, 0g protein

- *Truvia*

  - o Serving size: 1 packet; 0 calories, 0g fat, 3g carbs, <1g protein

- *JFC* White Shirataki Noodles (I recommend the 7oz pack to better keep track of the serving size)

  - o Serving size: ½ bag; 0 calories, 0g fat, 0g carbs, 0g protein

- *JFC* Brown Shirataki Yam Noodles (I recommend the 7oz pack again)

  - o Serving size: look on the bag; 5 calories, 0g fat, 2g carbs, 0g protein

- Eggs

  - o Serving size: 1 egg; 70 calories, 5g fat, 0g carbs, 6g protein

- Blueberries

  - o Serving size: ¼ cup; 20.75 calories, 0.13g fat, 5.25g carbs, 0.28g protein

- Mangoes

  - o Serving size: ½ cup sliced; 53.5 calories, 0.2g fat, 14.05g carbs, 0.4g protein

- Bananas (medium)

  - o Serving size: ½; 52.5 calories, 0.2g fat, 13.5 carbs, 0.65g protein

- Pineapples

  - o Serving size: 1 cup diced; 78 calories, 0.2g fat, 20.3g carbs, 0.8g protein

- Apples (medium)

  - o Serving size: 1 apple; 95 calories, 0.3g fat, 25.1g carbs, 0.5g protein

- *Confucius* Shrimp Eggrolls

- - Serving size: 1 eggroll; 110 calories, 2g fat, 11g carbs, 10g protein
- Green Onions
  - Serving size: 1 cup chopped; 32 calories, 0g fat, 7g carbs, 2g protein
- Clementines
  - Serving size: 1 clementine; 35 calories, 0.1g fat, 8.9g carbs, 0.6g protein
- Celery
  - Serving size: 110g; 18 calories, 0g fat, 4g carbs, 1g protein
- Green Bell Pepper
  - Serving size: 1 pepper; 33 calories, 0g fat, 7.5g carbs, 1.5g protein
- Bok Choy
  - Serving size: 70g; 9 calories, 0g fat, 2g carbs, 1g protein
- Spinach
  - Serving size: 1 oz; 6 calories, 0g fat, 1g carbs, 1g protein
- Light Italian Dressing (Fat Free)
  - Serving size: 2 Tbsp.; 15 calories, 0g fat, 3g carbs, 0g protein
- Light Ranch dressing
  - Serving size: 2 Tbsp.; 80 calories, 7g fat, 3g carbs, 0g protein
- *Golden* Zucchini Pancakes
  - Serving size: 1 pancake; 70 calories, 3g fat, 8g carbs, 2g protein
- *Golden* Vegetable Pancakes
  - Serving size: 1 pancake; 70 calories, 3g fat, 10g carbs, 2g protein
- Whole Wheat *Ritz* Crackers
  - Serving size: about 5; 70 calories, 2.5g fat, 11g carbs, 1g protein
- Reduced Fat *Ritz* Crackers

- Serving size: about 5; 70 calories, 2g fat, 11g carbs, 1g protein

- *I Can't Believe It's Not Butter!* Fat free

  - Serving size: 14g; 5 calories, 0g fat, 0g carbs, 0g protein

- *I Can't Believe It's Not Butter!* Mediterranean Blend Light Spread with Olive Oil

  - Serving size: 14g; 50 calories, 5g fat, 0g carbs, 0g protein

- *I Can't believe It's Not Butter!* Sweet Cream and Calcium Spread

  - Serving size: 14g; 50 calories, 5g fat, 0g carbs, 0g protein

- *I Can't Believe It's Not Butter!* Light Spread

  - Serving size: 14g; 50 calories, 5g fat, 0g carbs, 0g protein

- Grapefruit

  - Serving size: ½; 41 calories, 0.1g fat, 10.3g carbs, 0.8g protein

- Stila Bits

- Stila fruit crisps

- Edamame

- Veggie burger

- Veggie Straws